Daniel Fast Diet

Step By Step Guide for Beginners

Including Breakfast, Dips, Smoothie, Breakfast, Lunch, Dinner, Snacks and Dessert Recipes!

Disclaimer

The ideas, concepts and opinions expressed in this book are intended to be used for educational purposes only. This book is provided with the understanding that authors and publisher are not rendering medical advice of any kind, nor is this book intended to replace medical advice, nor to diagnose, prescribe or treat any disease, condition, illness or injury.

It is imperative that before beginning any diet or exercise program, you receive full medical clearance from a licensed physician. Author and publisher claim no responsibility to any person or entity for any liability, loss, or damage caused or alleged to be caused directly or indirectly as a result of the use, application or interpretation of the material in this book.

Formed using guidelines given in the scriptures, the Daniel Fast diet is being popularly followed around the world by people who want to find health and spiritual peace at the same time. In this beginner's guide, you will learn everything you need to know about the Daniel Fast diet, including:

- What is Daniel Fast diet and why is it so popular?

- Health and Spiritual benefits of this diet

- Foods allowed on this fast diet

- A guide to planning your meals

- Recipes for Daniel Fast including breakfast recipes, lunch recipes, dinner recipes, snacks and desserts recipes

So, read on to find out how to achieve the best of physical and mental health using the Daniel Fast Diet in this step by step guide for beginners.

Table of Contents

Why Daniel Fast?

In this fast life, we have become so distracted by our daily routines, stresses and full schedules that we never find the time to return to our lord and seek for his guidance. As a result, we are depressed and we have lost peace of mind. Amongst this chaos, by following the 21 day Daniel Fast, we can turn our attention back to Our Lord for duration of 21 days, by giving up food that we find pleasure in and by praying excessively.

There are many benefits of the Daniel Fast, according to the followers of this fast, all over the world. For 21 days, by focusing on God and unloading all our troubles through prayer and sacrifice, we are purging our souls from the heavy load of troubles. Here is a short list of the many benefits one can reap from following a 21 day Daniel fast.

- Fasting and praying brings us back in sync with God, opening us to his guidance and allowing us to lead a life as guided by him. It brings us closer to our Lord and brings back our lost peace of mind and showers us with serenity.

- When we refrain from the food that our body craves, we seek to fulfill our hunger with prayers and thus we develop an adjustment in our attitudes so that we seek more of our lord every moment.

- It clears our mind, showers us in peace and opens our soul to spiritual breakthroughs.

- It induces a new discipline within our life, as we learn to control our desires, we learn self control which can be utilized in changing our lives and thus transforming ourselves into what we have always wanted to be. It also creates humbleness and humility in us which makes us more emphatic to other's pain and sorrow.

- We learn to shift our attitude from one of negativity to that of gratitude for all that our Lord has blessed us with. This allows us to tackle our battles better due to a more positive mindset.

- Apart from spiritual benefits, fasting has physical benefits as well. Returning spiritually to our Lord allows healing to take place within us, which helps rid us of many of the daily ailments that we suffer from due to over indulging in worldly desires. Fasting allows a natural healing to take place within us. Refraining from indulging in unhealthy and luxury foods stops the damage and allows healing to take place.

- It allows one to shed unwanted pounds, eliminate toxins, purify blood, increase energy, increase vitality and promote health of organs, and increasing the overall quality of one's life.

The concept behind the Daniel fast is shifting our attitude from that of worldly pleasure to that of God's presence. When we suffer during this fast, we seek help and guidance from the Lord in helping us stick with the fast and fight temptations, which brings us closer to God.

The Daniel Fast

All over the world, people are searching for happiness by working longer hours, believing that money can help them find happiness. In this endeavor, they are losing their health, peace of mind and losing sight of their priorities. Amidst this chaos, the Daniel Fast is a method of fasting that means to bring back a man's focus to what's important.

It is a technique that allows people the opportunity to search for happiness within them, instead of outside and helps them find spiritual peace. The background of the fast lies in the holy bible, and from it the basic structure of the fast has been extracted. Following the life of the prophet as described in scriptures, followers of the Daniel Fast are allowed to eat only vegetables, fruits and drink only water.

The Prophet didn't indulge in breads, fats, meats or sweeteners, which is why followers are not allowed to eat these as well, along with no processed or chemically treated food.

Eating this way allows us to forego the cravings of our flesh and learn to listen to our soul's needs instead. Eating in this healthy manner allows us to detox and heal our bodies, while soothing and healing our souls as well, finding satisfaction within us. *In the next chapter we will take a closer look at the foods we are allowed during these 21 days.*

Daniel Fast Food List

Fruits

The Daniel Fast allows consumption of all natural foods which includes all fruits in all forms.

Vegetables

The Daniel Fast allows consumption of all vegetables in all forms. However, deep fried vegetables are not allowed.

Whole grains

The Daniel Fast allows consumption of all whole grains such as; whole wheat pasta, brown rice, whole wheat bread and tortillas, rice cakes, millet, oats, quinoa, barley and popcorn.

Nuts and seeds

The Daniel Fast allows consumption of all nuts, nut butters and seeds. Refrain from overconsumption of these, though.

Legumes

The Daniel Fast allows consumption of all legumes, canned or dried. Due to their high protein content, these should be made a major part of every meal.

Oils

The Daniel Fast allows consumption of all quality oils.

Beverages

Only water is allowed.

Other Food Items Allowed

- Tofu
- Soy products
- Vinegar
- Seasonings

Foods Not Allowed

- Meat
- Chicken
- Animal Flesh of any kind
- All dairy Products
- Any kind of sweetener
- Bread of any kind
- Chemically treated or processed food
- Solid Fats
- All beverages other than water, including green tea and coffee

How to Follow Daniel Fast?

Within the Old Testament Book of Daniel, there are several recorded times when Prophet Daniel fasted to seek God's guidance and wisdom. During his fasting period, he experienced powerful visions that helped him become aware of what was to come and how to deal with them.

Within the Old Testament, there are accounts of Prophet Daniel's fasting, in which he gave up all delicacies, such as meat, wine and everything other than vegetables, fruits and water. Based on this fact, the Daniel Fast allows only these foods during the 21 days of fasting.

Keeping in mind that this was a partial fast, which allowed consumption of regular meals, the fast was in the form of refraining from delicacies, today the Daniel fast follows the same guidelines.

The only way a follower can stay strong and keep with the guidelines is by seeking Lord's guidance in fighting temptations and truly giving up the world by getting absorbed in prayers. As a result, the 21 day fast has to be followed along with regular extensive prayers throughout the day.

To focus on our prayers, we must first address what help we require from God and the purpose behind following this fast. Is it financial troubles, a health issue, a family member or anything else? During these 21 days, we must open our hearts and search our souls for answers to our problems through the help of our Lord.

As a result, of the guidelines in the Old Testament, there are no restrictions to how much food one can eat during the day. However, the purpose behind the fast is to struggle with the sacrifice and use it to bring ourselves closer to Our Lord, which is why it is advisable to stick with 3 main meals and 2 small snacks for a day.

All these meals must only comprise of the food items from the list of allowed food.

Daniel Fast Daily Plan

Eat three times daily, or less if you don't feel hungry. These meals can be any of the meals from the recipes given in the upcoming chapter. It is not necessary that you can prepare only dinner recipes at dinner time or lunch recipes at lunch times; any recipe can be used at any time of the day.

Drink as much water throughout the day as you can and eat as little as you can. Spend most times praying and seeking guidance from God.

The following are the requirements for the 21 day fast:

- No snacking or munching throughout the day, apart from the meal times and the 2 snacks allowed. When hungry, pray and seek solace in God.

- No sweets or junk food of any kind.

- Eat meals prepared using the food items on the allowed food list.

- No beverages of any kind, other than water.

- Pray during meals, before and after meals. Pray as many times as you can.

- In case you indulge in forbidden foods, seek Lord's forgiveness and get back on track. Increase your prayer time and intensity to ensure it doesn't happen again.

Daniel Fast Recipes

Breakfast, Dips and Smoothie Recipes

Home Made Mustard

Serves: 4

Cooking Time: 20 minutes

Ingredients

2 cups of white vinegar

2 onions, diced

1 teaspoon minced garlic

120 grams dry mustard

1 and half tablespoon oil

Salt as per taste

5 drops of Tabasco sauce

Recipe

In a medium saucepan, combine the first three ingredients.

Bring to boil and reduce heat to let it simmer for a further 5 minutes.

Remove from heat and transfer to a medium bowl and set aside to cool.

In the same saucepan, add mustard.

Once cooled, sieve the vinegar mixture into the saucepan with mustard.

Whisk well, and then add in seasonings.

On medium heat, cook the mixture until it is the consistency of mustard, while stirring constantly.

Cool before serving.

Banana Berry Smoothie

Serves: 2

Cooking Time: 10 minutes

Ingredients

1 cup liquid of your choice, such as water or nut milk

1 cup berries, frozen or fresh

1 large banana, sliced

Recipe

Combine all the ingredients in a blender.

Blend till smooth.

Pour into serving glasses and enjoy!

Faux Banana Milk Shake

Serves: 2

Cooking Time: 10 minutes

Ingredients

2 large banana, sliced

Half cup liquid of your choice, such as water or nut milk

Half cup of ice

Dash of cinnamon powder

Recipe

Combine all the ingredients in a blender.

Blend till smooth.

Pour into serving glasses and enjoy!

Date Honey Smoothie

Serves: 2

Cooking Time: 10 minutes

Ingredients

180 grams of tofu

Half cup liquid of your choice, such as rice or nut milk

Quarter cup of date honey

2 large banana, sliced

Quarter tablespoon of cinnamon powder

Dash of ground nutmeg

Recipe

Combine all the ingredients in a blender.

Blend till smooth.

Pour into serving glasses and enjoy!

Summer in a Bowl Salad

Serves: 4

Cooking Time: 20 minutes

Ingredients

450 grams of cooked black beans

3 large mangoes, diced

2 bell peppers, chopped

4 green onions, chopped

Quarter cup of cilantro, finely chopped

Quarter cup of lime or lemon juice

1 tablespoon oil

Tabasco sauce and salt to taste

Recipe

Combine all the ingredients in a large bowl and mix well.

Serve.

Morning Casserole

Serves: 2

Cooking Time: 20 minutes

Ingredients

1 tablespoon oil

1 onion, finely sliced

Half of a bell pepper, diced

1 cup tofu, diced

Salt to taste

Dried Oregano, Dried Basil, Rosemary and other Italian herbs for seasoning

Recipe

In a medium sauce pan or skillet, heat the one tablespoon of oil.

Add onions and fry till transparent.

Add bell peppers and fry for further two minutes.

Add the remaining ingredients and cook till vegetables are tender.

Serve and Enjoy!

Hummus

Serves: 4

Cooking Time: 10 minutes

Ingredients

6 teaspoons of lemon juice

1 tablespoon oil

450 grams of canned cooked black beans

1 teaspoon minced garlic

6 teaspoons of tahini

1 teaspoon of cumin powder

Salt and cayenne pepper to taste

Recipe

Add all the ingredients in a food processor, and process till smooth.

If liquid is desired to make processing easier, reserve a little of the liquid from canned beans and that half a teaspoon at a time until mixture is smooth.

Serve with sliced vegetables.

Tofu Scramble

Serves: 4

Cooking Time: 10 minutes

Ingredients

100 grams of firm tofu

1 medium zucchini, chopped

1 plum tomato, chopped

1 onion, chopped

1 bell pepper, chopped

2-3 spring onions, chopped

2 tablespoons of minced cilantro

1 teaspoon of garlic paste

Salt to taste

Pepper to taste

Recipe

Heat oil in a skillet and add all the ingredients to the pan.

Fry till tender.

Add seasonings and mix.

Serve and Enjoy!

Tofu Frittata

Serves: 4

Cooking Time: 65 minutes

Ingredients

Quarter cup or 4 tablespoons of olive oil

1 large onion, chopped

2-3 spring onions, chopped

4 cloves garlic, minced

2 teaspoon of garlic paste

2 potatoes, thinly shredded

Salt to taste

Pepper to taste

1 kg box of tofu

3 tablespoons of soy sauce

Recipe

In a medium sauce pan or skillet, heat one tablespoon of oil.

Add onions and fry till transparent.

Add in the chopped spring and fry another minute.

Mix in the garlic and sauté for another minute, before adding the potatoes.

On medium-high, let the potatoes fry for fifteen minutes, after adding in the salt and pepper, mixing frequently.

Add the tofu in a blender and add in dash of salt, soy sauce and pepper or as per your taste. Blend until smooth.

Add this mixture to potatoes when done. Mix well.

Take a pie dish and spoon the whole mixture into the dish.

Bake for 35 minutes or until firm.

Serve and Enjoy!

Apple Breakfast Porridge

Serves: 4

Cooking Time: 65 minutes

Ingredients

1 liter water

1 and half cups of oat bran

1 cup of diced apple

Half a cup of raisins

1 teaspoon ground cinnamon

Half a teaspoon of salt

Recipe

Take a large saucepan and add water to it, bring to boil.

When the water starts boiling, add the oat bran.

Over medium heat, let the oat bran cook, stirring frequently for approximately 2 minutes.

Turn off the stove and add the remaining ingredients, stirring frequently until apple reach desired softness.

Serve with preferred milk.

Lunch Recipes

Cashew Rice

Serves: 4

Cooking Time: 45 minutes

Ingredients

2 cups of sticky rice

1 can of coconut milk

Half cup of water

Salt to taste

1 tablespoon oil

2 large onions, sliced

1 cup of peas, prepared

Half a cup of cashew, toasted

Recipe

Rinse rice under water until clean.

In a saucepan, add rice, milk, seasonings and water.

Cook over medium heat until mixture boils. Once boiled, cover the pan and let the rice cook over low heat for twenty minutes.

When the time is up, give the mixture a stir, and cover and cook for additional fifteen minutes.

When all of the liquid is absorbed, mix in peas and cashews.

In another pan, heat oil and fry onions till caramelized and slightly crispy.

Serve the rice with onions.

Baked Tofu

Serves: 2

Cooking Time: 45 minutes

Ingredients

200- 240 grams of firm tofu

Quarter cup of natural pineapple juice

3 tablespoons soy sauce

1 teaspoon minced garlic

Recipe

Chop the tofu in bite sized cubes and place them in a square baking dish.

The next step is preparing a marinade for the tofu, using the remaining ingredients. Combine all ingredients and mix well.

Add this mixture to the baking dish and coat tofu well. Set aside for 40 minutes.

Place the dish in a pre heated oven and bake for 20 minutes, until tofu is golden in color. Preheat oven to 350 degrees.

Beans and Rice

Serves: 4

Cooking Time: 15 minutes

Ingredients

1 tablespoon oil

1 onion, finely sliced

Half of a bell pepper, diced

3 celery, chopped

Quarter cup of water

450 grams of kidney beans

2 cups of brown rice, prepared

One third of a tablespoon paprika powder

Quarter teaspoon of onion powder

Quarter teaspoon of garlic powder

Dash of salt

Dash of pepper

Dash of thyme

Dash of dried basil

Dash of dried oregano

Dash of cayenne pepper

Recipe

Over medium heat, heat oil in a saucepan.

Add all the vegetables in the pan and cook until tender.

Next add the water and all the seasonings. Mix well.

Add in beans. Mix and add rice.

Cook on reduced heat for 5 to 8 minutes, until done.

Serve.

Bean Chili

Serves: 6

Cooking Time: 25 minutes

Ingredients

1000 grams of kidney beans

2 cups of brown rice, prepared

500 grams canned tomato sauce

250 grams of canned corn

1 cup of chopped bell peppers, roasted

1 onion, chopped

3 teaspoon of chili powder

Recipe

In a medium sized bowl, add beans and mash them. In to the mashed beans, add all the vegetable and seasonings.

Prepare a rectangular baking dish by rubbing with oil and pre heat oven for 12 minutes.

Place the casserole in the oven, after adding the mixture to it.

Bake for 20 to 25 minutes

Serve!

Wild Rice

Serves: 4

Cooking Time: 15 minutes

Ingredients

Half a cup of kidney beans

2 cups of brown rice, prepared

1 cup of chopped bell peppers, roasted

1 onion, chopped

1 tablespoon oil

1 onion, finely sliced

200 grams of chopped canned pineapple and juice

2 tablespoons soy sauce

1 teaspoon minced garlic

1 tablespoons lemon juice

2 large carrots, sliced

1 cup of peas

1 cup of zucchini, diced

Half a cup of canned chickpeas

Avocado slices and nuts for garnishing

Recipe

In a medium sauce pan or skillet, heat one tablespoon of oil.

Add onions and fry till transparent.

Mix in the garlic and sauté for another minute.

Add juices and soy sauce, mix well.

Stir in the remaining ingredients, except rice and pineapple bits.

Over medium heat, cook the mixture, stirring often, until liquid evaporates and vegetables are tender.

Mix in the rice and pineapple bits and stir fry for a few minutes until mixture is heated through.

Serve!

Spinach Casserole

Serves: 4

Cooking Time: 45 minutes

Ingredients

800 grams of canned tomatoes

1 teaspoon of garlic paste

1 teaspoon of salt

Dash of pepper

2 teaspoon of dried basil

2 teaspoon of oregano

2 teaspoon of dried parsley

3 zucchini, sliced

3 cups of spinach leaves

2 onions, sliced

Cooked brown rice

Recipe

In a medium sized saucepan, add seasonings and tomatoes.

Cook till mixture starts boiling.

Once boiled, reduce heat and let simmer for 12 minutes.

Prepare a rectangular baking dish by rubbing with oil and pre heat oven for 12 minutes.

Place zucchini in a layer in the dish.

Top the zucchini layer with a layer of spinach leaves and onions.

Pour the sauce over this mixture, when the tomatoes are cooked through and resemble pasta sauce.

Bake for 20 to 25 minutes

Serve with rice!

Vegetable Stew

Serves: 4

Cooking Time: 55 minutes

Ingredients

6 teaspoons of oil

1 cup of onions, diced

500 grams of string beans

500 grams of fresh spinach

1 liter of water

5 medium zucchini, chopped

3 squash, chopped

3 cups celery

2 cups of chopped tomatoes

Salt to taste

2 lemons, sliced

6 teaspoons of dried oregano leaves

6 teaspoons of dried basil

1 tablespoon of minced garlic

6 teaspoons lemon juice

Recipe

In a medium sauce pan or skillet, heat two tablespoon of oil.

Add onions and fry till transparent.

Mix in the oregano and garlic and sauté for another minute.

Pour in the water and mix well.

Add in the tomatoes and mix.

Cook for a further 12 minutes, stirring occasionally.

Mix in the remaining vegetables and seasonings.

Cover the pan and let cook for a further 40 minutes, stirring often.

Serve after topping with lemon slices.

Vegetable Stew with Rice

Serves: 4

Cooking Time: 55 minutes

Ingredients

200- 240 grams of firm tofu

Quarter cup of natural pineapple juice

3 tablespoons soy sauce

1 teaspoon minced garlic

1 teaspoon minced ginger

6 teaspoons of oil

1 cup of onions, diced

2 cups of broccoli

3 medium carrots, chopped

1 tablespoon tahini

Quarter cup of natural pineapple juice

2 cups of cooked brown rice

Quarter cup of walnuts, chopped and toasted

Sesame seeds for garnish

Recipe

Chop the tofu in bite sized cubes and place them in a square baking dish.

The next step is preparing a marinade for the tofu, using the remaining ingredients. Combine all ingredients and mix well.

Add this mixture to the baking dish and coat tofu well. Set aside for 40 minutes.

Drain the marinade (reserving the liquid for use later), but leave the tofu in the dish.

Place the dish in a pre heated oven and bake for 20 minutes, until tofu is golden in color. Preheat oven to 350 degrees.

When the tofu is done baking, take a large sauce pan or skillet, and heat two tablespoon of oil in it.

Add onions and fry till transparent.

Mix in the reserved marinade, and mix well.

Add the tofu, vegetables, ginger and garlic, mix well.

Cover and cook for ten minutes, stirring occasionally.

Mix in the juice and rice, along with nuts and mix well.

When the rice is heated through and juice is absorbed, mix in seeds and serve.

DIY Tortillas

Serves: 8

Cooking Time: 55 minutes

Ingredients

1 cup of warm water

2 cups of flour, whole wheat

Half a cup of soy flour

1 teaspoon of salt

Recipe

Mix all the ingredients together and knead until a ball is formed from the dough.

Transfer the dough to a work surface. Make sure it is dusted with flour to make kneading and working with it easier.

Knead for a further 5 minutes.

Place the dough in to a bowl and cover with plastic. Leave for 30 minutes in the same room.

Take the dough and divide it in eight balls.

Roll out each ball to form a tortilla with a 4 inch diameter and a thickness of a quarter inch.

Take a skillet and lightly spray it with oil. Heat it on medium flame.

Place the tortilla on the pan and cook it for a minute, before turning over to the other side.

Cook for a further two minutes.

Remove and set it on a plate and continue cooking the remaining tortillas similarly.

Serve with filling of your choice.

Greek-Style Stuffed Peppers

Serves: 8

Cooking Time: 55 minutes

Ingredients

1 teaspoon minced ginger

6 teaspoons of oil

1 cup of onions, diced

1cup zucchini, chopped

500 gram can of tomato sauce

6 canned artichokes, diced

1 cup of black olives, sliced

1 tablespoon of oregano flakes

1 tablespoon of parsley flakes

1 teaspoon salt

8 large bell peppers, de-seeded and tops cut off, to fill

4 cups quinoa, cooked

4 tablespoons pine nuts or any nuts

Recipe

Preheat oven for 12 minutes at 350 degrees.

Take the canned artichokes and place them in a food processor.

Pulse the artichokes until ground.

Take a large sauce pan or skillet, and heat oil in it.

Add onions and zucchini in the pan and fry till onions are transparent.

Reduce heat and add minced garlic to the pan.

Stir and cook for a further 1 minute.

Mix in all the other ingredients apart from the peppers.

Cook for 15 to 20 minutes, until the sauce reaches desired consistency.

Add in the quinoa and nuts.

Remove from heat.

Take the bell peppers and boil them in water for five minutes.

Remove and drain the bell peppers and place them in a rectangular baking dish.

Spoon this mixture into the bell peppers evenly.

Fill the dish with water till it reaches a height of half an inch.

Place in the oven and bake for 20 to 25 minutes.

Serve!

Dinner Recipes

Garlicky Peas

Serves: 8

Cooking Time: 25 minutes

Ingredients

1 and a half liter of water

1 kilo peas

2 tablespoons of oil

1 cup of chopped leeks

1 tablespoon of ground garlic

1 teaspoon salt

Half teaspoon pepper

Recipe

Pour the water in a pan over medium heat. When it is boiling, add in the peas and place the lid on the pan.

After five minutes reduce the heat and simmer for a further 5 minutes.

In a separate pan, heat oil and add garlic and leeks. Stir fry for a further 3 minutes.

When peas are done, drain and stir in the garlicky leeks, salt and pepper.

Mix well and serve!

Falafel

Serves: 8

Cooking Time: 40 minutes

Ingredients

400 grams canned chickpeas

Half a cup of brown rice flour

1 diced onion

2 teaspoons of dried parsley

2 tablespoons of oil

2 tablespoons of water

1 teaspoon minced garlic

Half a teaspoon of ground cumin

Pinch of salt

Pinch of cayenne pepper

Quarter cup of tahini

Quarter cup of lemon juice

Recipe

Preheat oven for 12 minutes at 325 degrees.

In a food processor, add flour, chickpeas, onion, parsley, oil, water, garlic, cumin, salt and pepper. Pulse till the consistency of a thick paste is achieved.

Use quarter cup of the paste to form a round ball.

Flatten the ball slightly. Continue making patties out of the entire mixture.

Place the patties on a baking sheet and bake for fifteen minutes and then flip and bake for a further fifteen minutes on the flip side.

In a small bowl, mix together tahini and lemon juice.

When falafels are done, take them out and serve by placing each falafel inside a whole wheat tortilla or half a whole wheat pocket bread, topped with lemon and tahini sauce. Add chopped vegetables of your choice.

Baked Kale with Beans

Serves: 5

Cooking Time: 70 minutes

Ingredients

Squash weighing approximately a kilogram

1 tablespoon oil

2 onions, chopped

1 teaspoon minced garlic

Half a cup of vegetable broth

400 grams of canned beans, drained

4-5 cups of kale, chopped

2 pinches of dried thyme

1 teaspoon of dried parsley

Recipe

Preheat oven for 12 minutes at 325 degrees.

Wash and clean the squash and then slice the squash in half, slicing it lengthwise.

Scoop out the seeds so that there is a hollow inside the vegetable.

Place the squash in a baking dish, filled with water to about quarter inch depth.

Bake the squash for 40 minutes.

When done, remove from the dish and let cool.

In a pan, heat oil and fry onions till they are transparent.

Add garlic to the pan and sauté for half a minute. Add in the broth, vegetables and seasonings. Mix and place the lid on the pan. Let the contents of the pan cook for 5 minutes.

If the squash has cooled down, skin it and chop it into bite size pieces.

Add the squash to the pan and continue cooking for 5 more minutes.

Serve!

Lentils

Serves: 6

Cooking Time: 40 minutes

Ingredients

750 ml of water

1 cup of brown lentils, rinsed

One third of a tablespoon paprika powder

Quarter teaspoon of onion powder

Quarter teaspoon of garlic powder

Dash of salt

Dash of pepper

Dash of thyme

Dash of dried basil

Dash of dried oregano

Dash of cayenne pepper

1 tablespoon of oil

2 medium onions, sliced

3 cups of brown rice, prepared

Recipe

In a medium saucepan, add in water and lentils. Let the mixture boil.

Once a boil is achieved, reduce heat and add in all the seasonings.

Mix and place the lid on the pan. Let the contents of the pan cook for 40 minutes until almost all water is absorbed and lentils are done.

In a separate saucepan, heat oil and add onions to it. When onions are caramelized and dark brown in color, remove the pan from the stove.

When lentils are done, remove the lid and pour the onions with oil on the lentils.

Replace lid and let stay for five minutes.

Serve with rice.

Quick Chickpea Casserole

Serves: 6

Cooking Time: 40 minutes

Ingredients

Half a cup of water

1 and a half cup of spinach leaves, cooked and drained

2 zucchini, chopped

2 carrots, chopped

2 spring onions

Pinch of salt

2-3 cups of brown rice, cooked

6 teaspoons of lemon juice

1 tablespoon oil

450 grams of canned cooked black beans

1 teaspoon minced garlic

6 teaspoons of tahini

1 teaspoon of cumin powder

Salt and cayenne pepper to taste

Recipe

Add lemon juice, oil, canned chickpeas, garlic, tahini, cumin and salt and cayenne into a food processor, and process till smooth.

If liquid is desired to make processing easier, reserve a little of the liquid from canned beans and that half a teaspoon at a time until mixture is smooth.

Preheat oven for 12 minutes at 325 degrees.

Add into the chickpeas mixture, water, vegetables, salt and rice. Mix well.

Spoon this mixture into a baking dish, pre-rubbed with oil.

Bake for 15 to 20 minutes.

Serve!

Vegetable Soup

Serves: 6

Cooking Time: 60 minutes

Ingredients

6 cups of water

2 celery, chopped

2 carrots, chopped

2 onions, chopped

1 teaspoon of salt

1 tablespoon oil

1 teaspoon minced garlic

450 grams of canned cooked black beans

250 grams of canned tomato sauce

450 grams of canned red kidney beans

450 grams of canned black-eyed peas

450 grams of canned green beans

1 cup of chopped squash, yellow

1 and a half teaspoon of chili powder

A dash of ground black pepper

Chopped parsley

Recipe

In a large saucepan, heat oil and add onions.

Mix in carrots and celery. Let the vegetables cook until tender.

Mix in minced garlic and stir for a minute.

Add in the remaining ingredients and let the mixture boil.

Once a boil is achieved, let the soup simmer for half an hour.

Garnish with parsley and serve!

Daniel Fast Frittata

Serves: 4

Cooking Time: 40 minutes

Ingredients

4 tablespoons of olive oil

Half a cup of onions, chopped

2 spring onions, chopped

2 teaspoons of minced garlic

2 cups of shredded potatoes

1 teaspoon salt

2 dashes of ground black pepper

1 kilogram tofu

3 tablespoons of soy sauce

1 teaspoon salt

Recipe

Preheat oven for 12 minutes at 325 degrees.

In a large saucepan, heat oil and add onions. Fry for 3 to 4 minutes until translucent.

Add in minced garlic and sauté for a minute, stirring constantly.

Mix in potatoes, a teaspoon of salt and add a dash of pepper to the pan.

Cook on medium high for 15 further minutes, stirring frequently.

In a food processor, mix tofu, a dash of pepper, soy sauce and a teaspoon of salt, blend until creamy.

Mix in the spring onions along with tofu mixture into the potatoes.

Pour the entire mixture into an oiled pie pan.

Place the pan into an oven and bake for 40 minutes. When the pie is done, the centre will be firm to touch.

Cool for ten minutes and then serve!

Potato Casserole

Serves: 4

Cooking Time: 50 minutes

Ingredients

6 tomatoes, chopped

5 potatoes, peeled and chopped

2 onions, chopped

Half a cup of olive oil

1 teaspoon dried parsley flakes

1 teaspoon dried basil flakes

1 and a half tablespoon dried oregano

120 ml of water

Half teaspoon powdered paprika

Half a tablespoon of salt

1 teaspoon black pepper

4 cups of tofu, cubed

Recipe

Preheat oven for 12 minutes at 325 degrees.

In a large bowl, combine all the ingredients and mix well.

Place in a baking dish and bake for 40-45 minutes.

Serve!

Vegetable balls

Serves: 4

Cooking Time: 150 minutes

Ingredients

1 cup of lentils, rinsed

3 cups of Broth

2 medium onions, chopped

2 teaspoon minced garlic

1 tablespoon oil

2 cups of button mushrooms, chopped

300 gram pack of frozen spinach

1 cup of brown rice flour

5 tablespoons of chopped nuts

2 teaspoon dried parsley flakes

2 teaspoon dried basil flakes

1 teaspoon garlic powder

1 teaspoon salt

Recipe

Preheat oven for 12 minutes at 325 degrees.

In a medium sized saucepan, add lentils, broth, half of the onions and garlic. Bring to a boil.

Once boiled, reduce heat and place lid.

Simmer for 45 minutes.

In a separate skillet, heat oil and add remaining onions and mushroom. Cook for two minutes and then add in spinach and cook for further three minutes, stirring.

Combine the two mixtures when lentils are cooked.

Mix in the remaining ingredients.

Process the entire mixture in a food processor until smooth.

Form balls and place on a lightly oiled baking dish.

Bake for 30 minutes.

Serve!

Bean Burgers

Serves: 6

Cooking Time: 50 minutes

Ingredients

400 grams of canned black beans

1 large or two medium sweet potatoes, mashed

Quarter cup of oats, grinded to form flour

1 and a half teaspoon parsley flakes

Two dashes of paprika powder

Two dashes of garlic powder

Two dashes of salt

Two dashes of pepper

Recipe

Mash three quarters of the beans, and leave the rest whole.

Mix in the rest of the ingredients.

Shape and flatten into burger patties and place them on an oiled baking sheet.

Broil in an oven for 8 minutes.

Flip burgers and broil for 3 more minutes on the other side.

Serve!

Snack Recipes

Almond Bites

Serves: 12

Cooking Time: 30 minutes

Ingredients

1 cup of almond butter

Half a cup of sunflower seeds

Half a cup of raisins

Half a cup of chopped almonds

5 tablespoons of shredded coconut, unsweetened

2 pinches of ground cinnamon

Recipe

In a medium sized bowl, combine butter, nuts, raisins, seeds, coconut and cinnamon. Mix well.

Form small balls and place on a baking dish.

Freeze till firm.

Ready to eat!

Almond Biscuits

Serves: 12

Cooking Time: 25 minutes

Ingredients

Half a cup of ground almond

One third of a cup of almond butter

Quarter cup of orange juice, unsweetened

7 tablespoons of Date Honey

3 tablespoons of slivered almonds

Recipe

Preheat oven for 12 minutes at 325 degrees.

In a large bowl, mix together all the ingredients, except honey and slivered almonds.

Knead or mix till a dough forms.

Prepare a baking dish by rubbing it with oil.

Spread the dough on a clean surface and cut out cookies.

Spread date honey on each cookie and place two to three slivered almonds.

Place the cookie sheet in oven and bake for 10-12 minutes.

Remove cookies and let cool before serving!

Apple Cookies

Serves: 12

Cooking Time: 25 minutes

Ingredients

3 small apples, peeled and chopped

1 cup of brown rice grinded to flour

1 cup of chopped walnuts or cashews

1 cup of pecans

1 cup of raisins

Recipe

Preheat oven for 12 minutes at 325 degrees.

In a large bowl, mix together all the ingredients.

Transfer the mixture to a food processor and process till smooth.

Drop spoonfuls of the mixture on a lightly oiled baking sheet, keeping about 5 cm distance between them.

Place the cookie sheet in oven and bake for 10-12 minutes.

Remove cookies and let cool before serving!

Kale Chips

Serves: 12

Cooking Time: 25 minutes

Ingredients

6 cups of kale leaves, torn into small bites

1 tablespoon of oil

2 pinches of garlic powder

2 pinches of salt

Recipe

Preheat oven for 12 minutes at 325 degrees.

Prepare a baking dish by rubbing it with oil.

In a large bowl, mix together all the ingredients until kale is completely coated.

Place the leaves on the baking dish.

Place the dish in oven and bake for 10-12 minutes, until crispy.

Serve!

Date Honey

Serves: 12

Cooking Time: 60 minutes

Ingredients

1 cup of dates, pits removed

250 ml of water

2 pinches of ground cinnamon

Recipe

In a medium sized saucepan, add the water and dates.

Bring the mixture to a boil.

Once boil is achieved, reduce the heat and let the dates cook for 60 minutes.

Remove the pan from stove and leave to cool.

Pour this mixture into a food processor and pulse until smooth.

Mix in cinnamon and store in an air tight container.

Fruit Bars

Serves: 12

Cooking Time: 20 minutes

Ingredients

2 large bananas, sliced

1 cup dates, chopped

1 cup cashews, chopped

Recipe

Place the three ingredients in a food processor and pulse until smooth.

Pour this mixture into a lightly oiled baking dish.

Freeze for 4 hours, until completely firm.

Once frozen, cut into bars and serve.

Daniel Fast Healthy Granola

Serves: 6

Cooking Time: 20 minutes

Ingredients

Quarter cup of dried dates

Quarter cup of water

1 cup of oats

One eighth of a cup of natural apple juice

1 tablespoon of oil

Quarter cup of raisins

One eighth of a cup almonds, chopped

One eighth of a cup walnuts, chopped

One eighth of a cup sunflower seeds

One eighth of a cup shredded coconut, unsweetened

Recipe

Preheat oven for 12 minutes at 325 degrees.

In a medium sized saucepan, add dates and water. Bring to a boil and then leave to cook for 5 to 5 minutes until softened.

Pour this mixture into a food processor and pulse until smooth.

In a larger bowl, combine all the ingredients along with date paste. Mix well.

Spread this mixture onto a lightly oiled baking dish or sheet.

Place the dish in oven and bake for 5 minutes.

Give it a good stir and bake for another 5 minutes

Let cool before serving.

Sesame Seed Crackers

Serves: 6

Cooking Time: 20 minutes

Ingredients

1 cup of brown rice, cooked

1 cup of brown rice ground to a flour

Quarter cup of flax seeds, ground

4 tablespoons of water

One eighth of a cup of oil

1 teaspoon of salt

1 teaspoon each of black sesame seeds and white sesame seeds

Recipe

Preheat oven for 12 minutes at 325 degrees.

Combine all ingredients together except the seeds.

Transfer this mixture into a food processor and pulse until smooth.

Pour this mixture into a bowl and add in seeds. Mix well.

Roll this dough using a rolling pin, wide enough to fit into a baking dish.

Place this rolled out dough into a lightly oiled 11 x 17 inch baking dish.

Place the dish in oven and bake for 10 minutes.

Keep removing squares that are done and leave the ones that require more baking until each piece is removed.

Serve!

Trail

Serves: 6

Cooking Time: 5 minutes

Ingredients

1 cup of almonds

1 cup of cashew pieces

1 cup of chopped walnuts

1 cup of raisins

2 tablespoons of sunflower seeds

2 tablespoons of pumpkin seeds

Recipe

Mix together all the ingredients and use 2 tablespoons of this mixture to snack on.

Pecan Stuffed in Dates

Serves: 4

Cooking Time: 5 minutes

Ingredients

8 dates, pitted

4 pecans, halved

Recipe

Stuff each pecan half inside a date.

Stuff all the dates.

Serve!

Dessert Recipes

Baked Apples

Serves: 4

Cooking Time: 25 minutes

Ingredients

3 apples, sliced

1 and a half cup of natural apple juice

2 pinches of ground cinnamon

Recipe

Preheat oven for 12 minutes at 325 degrees.

Place apples in a baking dish.

In a bowl, mix together apple juice and ground cinnamon.

Pour this mixture over apples.

Place the dish in oven and bake for 15 minutes.

After 15 minutes, give the apples a good stir and bake for a further 15 minutes.

Serve!

Avocado Gelato

Serves: 4

Cooking Time: 35 minutes

Ingredients

3 avocados, peeled and chopped

Quarter cup of coconut butter

Quarter cup of date honey

Quarter cup of sugar-free, protein powder, chocolate

One- eighth of a cup of unsweetened dark cocoa powder

Half a cup of natural almond milk, sugar-free

Quarter cup of coconut flakes, sugar-free, natural

Recipe

In a blender, add honey, avocados, butter, protein powder, cocoa powder and milk.

Blend well until smooth.

Lightly oil a cookie sheet.

Drop tablespoons of mixture onto cookie sheet, in ball shape.

Sprinkle the mixture with coconut flakes.

Place cookie sheet in freezer and freeze for 3 hours until solid.

Serve once frozen.

Apple Cobbler

Serves: 6

Cooking Time: 45 minutes

Pie Crust

Ingredients

2 cups walnuts, chopped

Half a cup of honey

3 teaspoons of ground cinnamon

2 additional teaspoon of cinnamon powder

1 teaspoon of sea salt

Recipe

In a grinder or food processor, grind the nuts till completely floured.

Next mix in cinnamon and salt and grind once more.

Next add honey and process until the mixture takes shape of a dough ball.

Take the dough and spread it in a pie dish.

Refrigerate for 15 minutes while preparing the topping.

Topping

Ingredients

4-5 cups of chopped or sliced apples

Quarter cup of agave or honey

3 teaspoons of ground cinnamon

1 teaspoon of ground nutmeg

A pinch of sea salt

Recipe

In a large bowl, add apples and mix in spices.

Combine to coat well.

Mix in sweetener and once again mix well.

Leave the mixture for an hour, allowing the juices and flavors to blend.

Add the topping into the prepared crust.

Bake for 20 minutes until apples are tender.

Serve Warm.

Oat Bars

Serves: 14

Cooking Time: 45 minutes

Ingredients

2 cups of rolled oats

Half a tablespoon of baking powder

2 generous pinches of salt

1 tablespoon of ground cinnamon

Stevia or honey as per taste

1 cup of coconut milk, low fat or non fat

Egg substitute equivalent to one egg

Half a cup of sugar-free applesauce

2 teaspoons of vanilla essence

1 cup of chocolate chips, dairy-free

Recipe

Preheat oven for 12 minutes at 350 degrees

Prepare a baking pan by lightly coating with oil.

In a food processor, add oats, egg substitute, salt, cinnamon and baking powder.

Process to mix well.

Next add in the sweetener, applesauce, vanilla and milk.

Mix well to thoroughly combine all ingredients.

Fold in chocolate chips.

Pour this mixture into the pan.

Place the pan into the oven.

Bake for 30 minutes.

Remove from oven, when done, and cut into squares.

Serve.

Chewy Oaties

Serves: 8

Cooking Time: 35 minutes

Ingredients

Quarter cup of organic butter

Quarter cup of sugar

Egg substitute equivalent to 2 egg whites

Three-quarters of a cup, unsweetened applesauce

Quarter cup of concentrated apple Juice

Half a tablespoon of Vanilla extract

Three-quarters of a cup flour

Quarter cup of whole wheat flour

1 teaspoon of baking soda

1 teaspoon of ground cinnamon

2 pinches of salt

1 and a half cup of rolled oats

Half a cup of raisins

Half a cup of chopped walnuts

1 tablespoon of sugar

Recipe

Preheat oven for 12 minutes at 325 degrees.

In a large mixing bowl, beat butter and sugar together.

Add in egg substitute, applesauce, juice and vanilla.

Whisk the mixture until thoroughly combined and smooth.

Mix in flours, soda, salt and cinnamon.

Beat until smooth.

Mix in oats, nuts and dried fruit.

Once again whisk the mixture until smooth.

Drop teaspoonfuls of the mixture on to a cookie sheet.

Place in the oven and bake for 15 minutes.

Once cooled, dust with sugar and serve.

Iced Coffee

Serves: 3

Cooking Time: 10 minutes

Ingredients

Quarter cup of sugar-free, protein powder, chocolate

1 banana, frozen earlier till completely solid

1 cup of ice

1 cup of almond milk

Recipe

In a blender, add all the ingredients and process till smooth.

Serve!

Chocolate Nut Bars

Serves: 5

Cooking Time: 25 minutes

Ingredients

4 bananas, frozen earlier till completely solid

One-eighth of a cup of peanut or almond butter

2 tablespoons of cocoa powder

1 tablespoon coconut butter

Quarter cup of coconut milk

Quarter cup of sugar-free, protein powder, chocolate

Sugar to taste

One-eighth of a cup of shaved coconut

Recipe

In a blender, add all the ingredients and process till smooth.

Top with shaved coconut.

Pour into serving moulds and place in freezer.

Freeze for 30 minutes.

Serve!

Chocolate Bark

Serves: 5

Cooking Time: 50 minutes

Ingredients

125 grams of chopped almonds

125 grams of chopped Macadamia Nuts

125 grams of chopped Hazelnut

125 grams of chopped Peanuts

125 grams of Pumpkin Seeds

125 grams of Sunflower Seeds

125 grams of Pistachios

1 kilogram of unsweetened dark Chocolate

Sugar to taste

Recipe

Preheat oven for 12 minutes at 325 degrees.

In a baking sheet, spread almonds evenly.

Add macadamia nuts and distribute evenly on the sheet.

Next add in the peanuts and distribute evenly onto the baking sheet.

Place the sheet in oven.

Bake for 15- 20 minutes.

The nuts should become golden in color.

Remove and transfer to a bowl.

In the same baking sheet spread pumpkin seeds evenly.

Add sunflower seeds and distribute evenly on the sheet.

Next add in the pistachios and distribute evenly onto the baking sheet.

Place the sheet in oven.

Bake for 10- 15 minutes.

The nuts should become golden in color.

Remove and transfer to a bowl.

When all the nuts and seeds have cooled down, spread them on a baking sheet lined with butter paper.

Pour melted chocolate over the nuts till completely coated.

Place in fridge, allow chocolate to cool.

Once completely cool, remove the butter paper and break it into pieces.

Store in an air tight container.

Brownies

Serves: 6

Cooking Time: 25 minutes

Ingredients

2 cups of walnuts

Half a cup of cocoa powder, unsweetened

One third of a cup agave or substitute that with 4 drops of stevia

One-eighth of a cup of peanut butter

3 teaspoons of cinnamon

1 teaspoon of sea salt

8 strawberries

Recipe

In a food processor, add cocoa, walnuts, peanut butter, salt, and cinnamon.

Process until completely combined.

Add in sweetener and continue processing until a ball of dough forms.

Transfer the mixture onto a pan and distribute evenly.

Cut into squares and serve!

Chocolate Cake

Serves: 7

Cooking Time: 45 minutes

Ingredients

Quarter cup of butter substitute

170 grams of Dark Chocolate, unsweetened

1 cup of walnuts or pecans

Dry egg substitute equivalent to 6 eggs

1 teaspoon of vanilla essence

Sugar to taste

1 pinch salt

Recipe

Preheat oven for 12 minutes at 325 degrees.

Prepare a baking pan by lightly oiling it.

Create a double boiler by placing a small saucepan over a large saucepan filled with simmering water.

Add chocolate in to the smaller saucepan along with butter substitute.

Stir constantly until chocolate has melted completely.

Let the chocolate cool.

In a food processor, grind the nuts until it is reduced to flour like consistency.

Mix in egg substitute and process once again.

Mix in vanilla and sugar. Process again until completely smooth.

Lastly mix in the chocolate and process again.

Pour batter into the prepared pan.

Bake for 30 minutes until toothpick comes clean when pierced in the centre of the cake.

Serve!

Chocolate Covered Bananas

Serves: 4

Cooking Time: 25 minutes

Ingredients

2 large bananas

225 grams of unsweetened dark chocolate

Half a cup of shaved coconut

Half a cup of almond slivers

Recipe

Slice bananas and insert a toothpick into each slice.

Arrange bananas on a baking tray after placing a sheet butter paper on it.

Create a double boiler by placing a small saucepan over a large saucepan filled with simmering water.

Add chocolate in to the smaller saucepan and keep stirring until completely melted.

Roll the banana slices in chocolate and roll in coconut and almonds.

Place them back on the sheet and continue coating banana until all slices are done.

Place the sheet into a freezer and freeze until completely solid, about an hour.

Serve!

Truffles

Serves: 7

Cooking Time: 25 minutes

Ingredients

Quarter cup of goji powder

Quarter cup of sugar-free, protein powder, chocolate

Half a cup of macadamia nuts

2 tablespoons of cocoa butter

Quarter cup of honey

10 drops of liquid stevia

Quarter cup of cocoa nibs

Quarter cup of chopped goji berries

Half a cup of coconut shavings

Recipe

Take a food processor and add goji powder and protein powder, along with nuts and process until mixed well.

Pulse a few more times.

Add in melted butter, honey and liquid stevia steadily in a slow trickle, do not add at once.

Blend further until the contents reach a creamy smooth consistency.

Add in the remaining ingredients and mix well using hand.

Shape into small balls and place on cookie sheet lined with parchment paper.

When all mixture is formed into balls, freeze.

Serve when firm.

Daniel Diet Smoothies

Cherry Banana Smoothie

Serves: 2

Cooking Time: 5 minutes

Ingredients

1 cup of coconut milk

1 large frozen banana

Half a cup of chopped cherries

1 tablespoon of chopped almonds

Recipe

Combine all the ingredients in a blender.

Blend till smooth.

Pour into serving glasses and enjoy!

Coconut Paradise

Serves: 2

Cooking Time: 5 minutes

Ingredients

Half a cup of water

Half a cup of coconut milk

1 cup of sliced frozen banana

1 cup of frozen blueberries

1 cup of frozen mango, chopped

1 cup of frozen chopped strawberries

Recipe

Combine all the ingredients in a blender.

Blend till smooth.

Pour into serving glasses and enjoy!

Plum Smoothie

Serves: 2

Cooking Time: 5 minutes

Ingredients

1 cup of cold water

1 medium chopped apple

1 cup of frozen chopped banana

Quarter cup of dried plums

1 tablespoon of ground flaxseed

1 tablespoon of coconut shavings

Recipe

Combine all the ingredients in a blender.

Blend till smooth.

Pour into serving glasses and enjoy!

Go Green Smoothie

Serves: 2

Cooking Time: 5 minutes

Ingredients

1 cup of almond milk

1 cup of kale and spinach leaves

1 cup of frozen chopped banana

Half a cup of frozen raspberries

One-eighth of a cup of chopped walnuts or pecans

Recipe

Combine all the ingredients in a blender.

Blend till smooth.

Pour into serving glasses and enjoy!

Spicy Banana Smoothie

Serves: 2

Cooking Time: 5 minutes

Ingredients

180 grams of firm tofu

Half cup of unsweetened soy milk

2 cups of sliced frozen banana

One-fourth of a cup of date honey

2 generous pinches of ground cinnamon

A dash of nutmeg

Recipe

Combine all the ingredients in a blender.

Blend till smooth.

Pour into serving glasses and enjoy!

Tangy Strawberry Smoothie

Serves: 2

Cooking Time: 5 minutes

Ingredients

120 grams of firm tofu

Quarter cup of unsweetened soy milk

Quarter cup of apple juice

One-eighth of a cup of date honey

1 cup of sliced or chopped frozen strawberries

1 cup of sliced frozen banana

Recipe

Combine all the ingredients in a blender.

Blend till smooth.

Pour into serving glasses and enjoy!

Mediterranean Smoothie

Serves: 2

Cooking Time: 5 minutes

Ingredients

1 cup unsweetened nut milk

1 cup of frozen sliced bananas

1 cup chopped frozen strawberries

1 date, pit removed

Recipe

Combine all the ingredients in a blender.

Blend till smooth.

Pour into serving glasses and enjoy!

Healthy Green Smoothie

Serves: 2

Cooking Time: 5 minutes

Ingredients

1 cup of unsweetened coconut milk

1 cup of frozen banana

1 cup of chopped frozen strawberries

1 cup of spinach and Kale leaves

6 teaspoons of ground flaxseed

Recipe

Combine all the ingredients in a blender.

Blend till smooth.

Pour into serving glasses and enjoy!

Strawberry Orange Smoothie

Serves: 2

Cooking Time: 5 minutes

Ingredients

1 cup of frozen strawberries

Half a cup of coconut milk

2 tablespoons of Honey

Quarter cup of fresh orange Juice

Recipe

Combine all the ingredients in a blender.

Blend till smooth.

Pour into serving glasses and enjoy!

Spinach Berry Smoothie

Serves: 2

Cooking Time: 5 minutes

Ingredients

1 cup frozen blueberries

230 grams of pure coconut water

1 and a half cup of baby spinach

2 tablespoons of chopped avocado

2 tablespoons of ground flax seeds

1 scoop of sugar-free, protein powder, chocolate

Few drops of liquid stevia

Recipe

Combine all the ingredients in a blender.

Blend till smooth.

Pour into serving glasses and enjoy!

Made in the USA
Las Vegas, NV
27 December 2023

83591588R00057